Bodyweight Training Guide

The Ultimate No Gym Workout Manual

Table of Contents

Introduction

I want to thank you and congratulate you for reading the *"Bodyweight Training Guide"*. This book contains proven steps and strategies on how to do bodyweight exercises and the results you desire.

Regular exercise is part of a healthy lifestyle but many people find excuses to avoid it. Whether you have a busy schedule or a tight budget, you can still reap the benefits of exercise by working out in the convenience of your own home.

Bodyweight exercises are done using your body as resistance. They can tone your body and increase your overall endurance and strength. Also, bodyweight exercises are perfect for people who do not feel comfortable at the gym. Most of these exercises do not require any equipment at all, although a few may need some form of leverage like a pole, a bar, or a wall. The main resistance in these exercises will be provided by your body. Another great thing about bodyweight exercises is that they can be performed both indoors and outdoors.

This book contains various exercises that target multiple muscle groups at the same time. You'll also find an 8-week sample exercise program for both beginner and advanced levels. You'll even learn how you can integrate cardio exercise into your routine. Additionally, you will find other helpful information about nutrition to improve your overall health and wellbeing.

Thanks again for reading this book, I hope you enjoy it and I wish you the best of success!

Mike

P.S. If you would like to check out some of my favorite bodyweight cross training exercises, visit: http://www.deepthoughtpress.com/bodyweight/

Chapter 1 Why Bodyweight Training?

Many people like the idea of being able to work out at their own homes. There are a lot of factors that prevent people from acquiring gym memberships. Bodyweight training is the most convenient type of resistance training. Below are some of the best benefits of bodyweight training.

It is very efficient

Studies show that people can still reap the benefits of exercise even if they do not go to the gym to work out. Performing high intensity bodyweight exercises can help your lose weight and tone your body even if you only exercise for a short amount of time. It is also easier to transition from one move to another since you do not use any equipment.

It combines strength training and cardio

One of the most common reasons why most people don't exercise is that they do not have enough time. You can still do cardio and strength training in one session. Quick bodyweight exercises like the burpees and jumping jacks can increase your heart rate and build muscles at the same time.

Good for everyone

Bodyweight exercise can be modified to suit your current fitness level. You can also add your own twist by adding extra repetitions or performing the exercise at different speeds.

Improved core strength

The core does not only pertain to the abs. It comprises of 29 muscles in the abdomen, lower back and butt. Many bodyweight exercises engage the core that can strengthen the muscles and even improve posture.

Better flexibility

Resistance training does not have to make your muscles sore. You can combine bodyweight and flexibility exercises. A bodyweight exercise that uses a full range of motion can lead to better posture and can reduce your risk of injury.

Convenience

Bodyweight is very convenient for everyone. You do not need any equipment nor do you need to spend a lot of time. Bodyweight exercises are easy to squeeze into your schedule.

Improved balance

Some bodyweight exercise like the pistol squat can increase body awareness and control. You can easily modify other exercises to make it more challenging. This is the reasons why bodyweight exercise is essential for improving athletic performance.

No more boredom

It can be very easy to get bored with a single exercise regimen. Incorporating different bodyweight exercises each time can be very refreshing and can spice up your workout. Bodyweight exercises also help prevent workout plateaus.

It is fun

Bodyweight exercises can be performed indoors or outdoors. You can also do it alone or practice with a group of friends. Bodyweight exercises can be fun and challenging at the same time.

Injury prevention

Injury can stop you from working out. It is essential that you take precautionary steps to prevent injury. Bodyweight exercises are deemed to be safe for everyone and some moves are even good for rehabilitation. Just make sure to spend a few minutes to warm up your muscles.

It is budget friendly

With so many advertisements on weight loss, many people seem to think that fitness comes at a high price. Buying equipment and enrolling in a gym can be expensive. Bodyweight exercises are free. You can also take advantage of your natural environment and exercise outdoors.

Delivers Results

Bodyweight exercise is effective because it integrates compound movements that engage large muscle groups and joints. These compound movements can help you improve your athletic performance.

Building the Body You Want Through Bodyweight Exercises

Although bodyweight training can provide you with great benefits on its own, you can incorporate bodyweight exercises into your regular fitness routine. Some athletes use bodyweight exercises as warm up, and body builders also try to integrate it between their weightlifting sessions. Here are some tips on how you can integrate bodyweight exercises to your routine:

Add it to your warm-up

Warm up is one of the most important parts of your workout. A good warm up can prepare your body for more strenuous exercise. Push-ups, squats and burpees are great warm-up exercises. This also allows you to build strength for heavy lifting and gives you the benefit of a good bodyweight exercise.

Learn several variations

Bodyweight exercise has many variations and modifying the moves can keep it challenging and fun. Once you feel that you have become better at one exercise, try other variations instead. As a start, you can devote 15 minutes of your fitness routine to bodyweight exercise.

Incorporate it in your cool down

You can perform a circuit of low impact bodyweight exercises as a cool down. This is also a great opportunity to integrate variations into your workout.

Bodyweight during your low-time

People who lift heavy weights or engage in high intensity workouts may need to rest in order to give the body enough time to recover. For most, it is not enough to rest for one day. You can schedule a few days to a few weeks of low impact and moderate intensity exercises. Bodyweight training is perfect for this resting phase. It enables you to continually strengthen your body without placing too much pressure on it. You can also adjust the duration of your workout if you need to.

Chapter 2 The Importance of Nutrition

The food that you consume provides your body with the needed energy to function. However, people eat food for a variety of reasons. People feel the urge to eat when they are hungry or tired. Other times, people can also use food for emotional reasons. People use food to celebrate happy occasion and to alleviate stress.

Nutrition provides raw materials for the body

Supplying the body with the essential macronutrients is essential for good health. Macronutrients comprises of protein, fat and carbohydrates. These are the main components of your diet. The human body also needs micronutrients like minerals and vitamins but in fewer quantities (compared to macronutrients).

Protein is broken down into amino acids that are used to repair tissues and promote muscle development. Muscles contain protein and you will need to continually supply your muscles with protein to avoid muscles loss. The most popular protein source is animal meat that also contains complete amino acids. Vegetarians can complete their daily protein requirement by combining legumes, beans and other vegetables.

Carbohydrate serves as the main fuel of the body. It can be tricky to know the right amount of carbohydrates that the body needs since consuming too many carbohydrates can lead to fat formation. Carbohydrates can either be simple or complex. Simple carbohydrates are beneficial for immediate energy consumption but complex carbohydrates supply the body with enough energy that can be used for a long period of time.

Fat is also essential for the body. It serves as the main insulator of the body and protects the organs from damage. The brain needs fatty acids and it is also used for hormone production.

Vitamins and minerals are just as important as macronutrients. They function as co-enzymes that speed up the chemical reactions in the body. Vitamin A helps improve vision, while Vitamin C keeps the immune system health. Your diet should contain a balanced amount of these nutrients.

<u>Tips on Nutritious Eating</u>

A balanced diet is not restrictive nor does it aim to deprive you of the food that you enjoy. A nutritious diet should make you feel more energized and happy. Here are some tips on how you can establish a nutritious diet:

Start slow and simple

Most people are overwhelmed about the information that they get about nutrition. Instead of eliminating a certain food group or counting calories, you can start by thinking about your food in terms of variety and freshness. Focus on finding healthy foods that you enjoy and incorporate them into your recipes. Changing your diet drastically overnight is not realistic. You can add small changes in your diet and it will become a habit over time.

Moderation is the key

Expecting that you need to eat 100% healthy all the time can only lead to disappointment and frustration. Eating in moderation means that you only eat as much as your body needs and not until your feel stuffed. You should also balance carbohydrates, protein and fat. The main goal of healthy eating is to make sure that you can sustain the diet for a long time.

You can still eat your favorite foods in moderation provided that your diet is generally healthy. You can also start adjusting your portion sizes. Remember that it doesn't take too much food to fill the stomach.

Change how you think about food

Healthy eating is more than placing food in your plate; it also involves the way you think about nutrition in general. Healthy eating habits can be developed over time.

- Take time to chew your food. This enables you to taste the flavor of the food better.
- Listen to your body. It can take some time before the body can realize that it is already full.
- Avoid eating at night. Eating an early dinner and fasting for around 14 hours can help your digestive system rest and may even regulate weight. If you must eat, opt for light and low fat snacks instead.

Eat the rainbow

Fresh fruits and vegetables come in different colors. The color of fruits and vegetables may indicate that they are rich in a particular nutrient. Aim to consume 5-7 servings of fresh produce every day. Greens are rich in zinc, vitamin A,E and K. Sweet vegetables like corn, onion and pepper add flavor to your dishes without adding unnatural ingredients. Fruits are called as nature's candy because they can curb your sweet craving and provide you with valuable nutrients.

Enjoy healthy carbs

Complex carbohydrates are rich in fiber. This type of carbohydrate can supply you with long lasting energy. It is also rich in antioxidants and phytochemicals. Studies show that people who consume more complex carbs have better heart health.

Enjoy healthy fat

Fat is essential to nourish the heart, brain and cells. Aim to consume food that is rich in omega 3 fatty acids that can improve your mood and prevent cardiovascular disease.

Limit sugar and salt

If the diet you consume is rich in vegetables, whole grains, protein and good fat, then you may observe that you are naturally reducing your sugar and salt intake.

Sugar can cause blood sugar spikes, which in turn can cause energy fluctuations. Sugar can also contribute to weight gain. You may be not be aware of the total amount of sugar you are consuming since sugar is present in almost all processed foods like bread, seasoning and liquid drinks. You can reduce sugar consumption by choosing naturally sweet foods (like fruits) instead.

Most people consume too much salt from processed foods and fast foods. Your daily sodium intake should be between 1,500 to 2,300 mg only which is equivalent to one teaspoon of salt. Reduce your salt intake by choosing fresh vegetables instead of canned goods.

Your taste buds may need some time to adjust to a low sugar and low sodium diet so it is better if you gradually reduce your seasoning.

Add calcium to your diet

Calcium is a key nutrient for the body. It is essential for maintaining good bone health. Make sure that you get your calcium from food instead of supplements as much as possible. Dairy products are rich in calcium that can easily be absorbed by the body. Green leafy vegetables and beans also contain calcium.

Chapter 3 Bodyweight Movements

Bodyweight exercises are great for a full body workout but you can also use it to target specific muscle groups in the body.

<u>Abdominal and Core Exercises</u>

The Plank

The plank is a great exercise for beginners. Begin by going on all fours and resting your weight on your forearm. Make sure to keep your torso straight and your neck should be relaxed. Pull your bellybutton in and hold the position.

Russian Twist

The Russian twist is great for the oblique muscles. Sit on the floor. You can plant you feet on the floor or raise it up for more challenge. Contract your abs and twist your torso to the right then left. You can also touch the floor as you rotate your body.

Alternating superman

Lie face down on the mat. Extend your arms above your head. Raise your left leg and right arm off the ground. Hold for a few seconds then repeat on the other side.

The Side Plank

The side plank can engage the lateral stabilizers that run from your shoulder to your ankle. This can also help strengthen the oblique and transverse. Lie on your right side then place your right forearm on the floor. Lift your body while keeping your spine straight.

V-sit

V-sit is a highly effective abdominal and core exercise that engages the abs and oblique. Start by sitting on the floor. Engage your abs and lift your left at a 45 degree angle. Extend your hand towards your leg. Make sure that your spine is straight. You can hold the position for a few seconds or make small pulsing movements.

Bicycle crunch

The bicycle crunch is one of the most popular exercises for the abs and oblique. Lie on the floor. Place your hand behind your head. Do not interlace your fingers to avoid straining your neck. Lift the knees at a 45-degree angle and push your legs in a pedaling motion. Touch your left elbow to your opposite knee and touch your right elbow to your left knee. This exercise should be preformed slow.

The hip bridge exercise

The hip bridge can target the abs and lower back muscles. Lay on your back. Place both arms on the sides. Bend your knees and keep your feet under your knees. Tighten the abs and glutes. Raise your hips off the floor. Engage your core for the entire duration of the exercise.

Skip Twist

This is a great warm-up exercise since it can raise your heart rate and engage large muscle groups at the same time. Start by slowly skipping for 10 counts. Stop then turn around. You can move faster with each round or add full arm swings.

Flutter kick

The quick movements of the flutter kick exercise can raise your heart rate while engaging your core. Lie on the floor and keep your arms at your sides. Your palms should be facing down. Raise your legs about 6 inches off the floor and perform up and down movements with your feet. Tighten your abdominals as you perform the exercise.

Sprinter sit-up

This is a quick exercise that can engage your core and legs. Lie on the floor and extend your legs straight. Bend your elbows in a 90-degree angle. Sit up then drive your left knee to the opposite elbow. Lower your hands and feet and repeat on the other side.

Chest and Back Exercises

Basic Push-up

This is one of the most popular bodyweight exercises because it is effective and simple. Start by placing your hands and feet in the floor. Your hands should be shoulder-width apart. Plant your feet at hip distance and engage your core. Lower your body and bend your elbows until you almost touch the floor. Push your body up and make sure to keep your elbow close to the body.

Donkey Kick

This bodyweight exercise can increase your heart rate and help tone your abs, chest and back. Begin in a plank position. Squeeze your core tight then kick both of your feet off the ground. Bend your knees and bring your feet to your glutes. Land softly in the starting position.

Judo Push-up

Judo push-up is a variation of the classic push-up. Begin in a push-up position with your feet slightly closer to your torso. Your hips should be raised to the ceiling. Use your arms to lower your torso until it almost touches the floor. Lift the shoulders and head up and hold the position for a second. Reverse the movement and return to the starting position.

Dolphin push-up

Dolphin push-up is more challenging than the basic push-up. It incorporates yoga and bodyweight exercise. Kneel down then lean forward. Place your elbows on the floor and place your elbows apart. Clasp your hands in front of you. Extend your legs behind you. Your body should look like an inverted V. Lower your head to your shoulders. Push your body up and return to the starting position.

Handstand push-up

The handstand push-up is a more advanced workout and should only be attempted by people who have successfully done a headstand. Start in a headstand position. You can do this against the wall. Bend your elbows to lower your body. This should look like an upside down push-up.

Reverse fly

The reverse fly can be done with or without weights. Start in a standing position. Place one foot in front of the other. Your front knee should be slightly bent. Close your hand in a fist and bring them together in front of you. Bend your torso forward and extend your arm to your sides. Make sure to squeeze your shoulder blades together.

Back extensions

Back extensions can be done with or without equipment. Lie face down on a bench. Have someone hold your feet then lift your torso up as far as you can go. Pause for a few seconds then lower your upper body.

Bird Dog exercise

The bird dog exercise also targets the lower back muscles. Start by going on your hands and knees. Place your hands below your hips. Lift your right hand and draw your left leg simultaneously. Make sure that both of your limbs are parallel to the floor. Pause for a few seconds then return to the starting position.

Biceps and Triceps Exercises

Knuckle Push-up

Knuckle push-up is a great variation to the basic push-up. This variation can be more comfortable if the regular push-up tends to strain your wrists. You will need to fold your hands into fists and perform the push-up with your knuckles. Your knuckles should be facing each other and your elbows should be kept close to your side.

Archer pull-ups

Archer pull-up is a great variation of the common pull-up. This exercise specifically targets the biceps. Grasp the pull-up bar or wall that is at least wider than shoulder-width. Pull your body to the left. Your right arm should be parallel to the bar overhead. Lower your body and repeat the same movement on the right.

Muscle-ups

Muscle-up is one of the exercises used in CrossFit. Basically, muscle-up is like transitioning from pull-up to a dip in one movement. Place your hand in a pull-up bar. Your thumbs should be on top of the bar and not wrapped around. Pull your body up until your chin is at the same level as the bar. Roll your chest over the bar. Grip the bar firmly then push your body upwards.

Chair dips

Chair dips can tone your triceps. Start by sitting at the edge of a chair. Place both hands at the edge of the seat. Keep your fingers pointing forward. Your feet should be together and bend your knees. Move your butt off the chair as you bend your elbows. Lower your body to the floor then push it back up.

Triceps extensions

Start by lying on your right side. Your feet should be stacked on top of each other. Place your right arm on your left shoulder and place your left hand on the floor near your chest. Push your body using your left triceps. Make sure that your hips and legs are straight. Lower your body to the starting position.

Reverse push-ups

A slight modification can turn an exercise for the biceps to one for the triceps. This exercise may seem unnatural at first but you will soon be comfortable with it as you progress. Place your hands farther than shoulder width apart. Turn your fingers outward to the side. It should be pointing towards the feet.

One arm push up

Push-ups can strengthen your biceps but after some time, you may find it too easy. Challenge your body by trying the one arm push-ups. This places the resistance on one arm and activates more muscle fibers. Start in a basic push-up position. Spread your legs wider than normal. Lift your hand off the floor and place it behind your back. Lower your body to the floor and push it back up using one arm. Switch hands and repeat the movements.

Decline push-up

Decline push-up is a great exercise for the upper body. Start in a push-up position and place your feet on top of stacked books or even a short chair. Perform the push-up and make sure to engage your abs through the movement.

Power punch

Boxing exercises are effective for toning the biceps and triceps. Stand with your feet apart. Move your right foot slightly forward. Ball your fingers into a fist then keep your elbows close to the body. Punch using the hand closest to your body. Make sure to rotate your torso as you punch. Switch sides and use your other hand to punch.

Uppercut

This is another great boxing move. Start in a fighting stance with one of your foot slightly forward. Bend your knees slightly as your drive your fist upwards, like you are aiming at the ceiling. Switch sides and repeat same movement.

Forearm Exercises

Wrist Curls

Wrist curls are one of the simple yet challenging exercises that can tone your forearms. Start by sitting in a chair or bench. Place your right forearm on your right leg and curl your fingers into a fist. Hold down your forearm using your other arm. Lift your right forearm against the resistance of your left arm. Repeat the movements on the other arm.

Wrist extensions

The wrist extension is a good strengthening and flexibility exercise. Hold your palms in front of you. Hold your fingers on the opposite hand and pull it back to the body. This movement should stretch your forearms. Hold the position for a few seconds then switch on the other arm.

Hammer curl

The hammer curl requires manual resistance and it is actually categorized as an isometric exercise. This means that the muscles contract but do not extend so the joints do not actually move. Stand straight then bend one of your arms into a 90-degree angle. Extend your fist in front of you. Your palms should be facing your body. Rest your other hand on top of your thumbs. Do not use too much pressure since this exercise should be done without joint movement. Hold the position for a few seconds then repeat the movement on the other arm.

Power Push-ups

Power training increases the amount of force exerted by your muscles in a short amount of time. This can also help you burn more calories per minutes. You can do a power push-up by simply increasing the speed of the movement. Push yourself as fast as you can as you push your hands off the floor. Land with your hands in the starting position.

Towel Wring-out

You can use simple household materials, like a towel, to target your forearms. This exercise may look simple but it is one of the most effective and convenient exercise for your forearms. Simply take a thick towel and soak it in water. Wring the towel to remove the excess water. Wring the towel in opposite directions. You may also opt to wring a dry towel but be sure to use force and resistance.

Shoulder Exercises

Pike push-up

The pike push-up can be adjusted to suit all fitness levels. This can also serve as training for people who wants to master the handstand push-up later on. Start in a push-up position. Make sure that your legs are straight. Walk your hands towards your feet until you are in a pike position. Your body should be in a 90-degree angle. Place both your hands overhead and make sure that it is in line with the spine. Keep your core engaged as you bend your elbows. Lower your body until your head is almost at the floor. Push your body back up and repeat the movement.

Shoulder rotation

The shoulder rotation is an exercise where you rotate your shoulders from your body. This exercise is also good for the core. Start in a plank position where you are resting on your elbows. Rest your body weight on your right elbow and rotate to the right side. Hold the position for a few seconds then return to the starting position but do not let your left elbow rest on the ground. Place it towards your right arm but do not let it touch the ground. This movement stretches the shoulder muscles. Rotate to a side plank before switching sides.

Crab walk

The crab walk may look childish but it can tone your shoulder and arm muscles. Start by sitting on the floor. Place your hands under your shoulder. Bend your knees and place your feet on the floor. Lift your hips a few inches off the floor. This is referred to as the crab pose. Walk forward using your feet and hands. Make sure that your opposite arm and leg is moving in tandem. Make sure that you keep your chest up.

Human flag

The human flag is an advanced move where your entire bodyweight is supported by your arms and shoulders. This exercise also targets the abdominals and back. Start by finding a pole and grip it firmly. Always ensure that the anchor point is stable. Make sure that your hands are perpendicular to the ground. Lift your outside leg first. This makes it easier to establish your position and balance. Use your lower arm as leverage as your lift your other leg. Your body should be raised horizontally.

Mountain Climbers

Mountain climber is a powerful full-body exercise. It can sculpt your core and shoulders. It is also beneficial for the legs and hips. Start in a push-up position. Make sure that your arms are below your shoulders. Squeeze your abs and drive your knee to your arm. Extend your leg back and repeat the same movement on the other knee. Do this as quickly as possible. Your feet should only touch the ground at the beginning of the exercise.

Hindu Push-ups

Hindu push-up is a comprehensive workout that targets the shoulders, chest and arms. Make sure that you are aware of your position at all times. Start in a push-up position. Lift your buttocks upward. Your legs should be farther apart. Your body should look like an inverted V. Keep your neck relaxed to reduce strain and pressure. Move your body down in a controlled motion. Your hips should move towards the floor while your head moves up. Slowly swing your body forward as you start to ascend so that you will end up arching your back. Once you are at the starting position, quickly do another repetition.

Leg Exercises

Wall sit

All you need for this exercise is your body and a wall as a guide. Stand in front of the wall and slide back down until you are parallel to the ground. Make sure to keep your spine straight. Your knees should be bent above your ankles. This will place resistance to your legs. Stay in the position for 5-15 seconds before standing up.

Squat

The squat is the most basic and most effective lower body exercise. It can tone your butt and sculpt your legs at the same time. Stand with your feet shoulder-width apart. You can clasp your hands in front of you or curl them into fists. Lower your hips until it is almost parallel to the floor. Your weight should rest upon your heels. Straighten your legs and squeeze your glutes at the end of the movement.

Lunge

Lunge is a great leg exercise that can be used as leg warm-up. Place your hands on your hips and keep your feet apart. Step the right leg forward and lower your torso. Bend your knees in a 90-degree angle. Straighten the legs and switch legs and repeat the same movements.

Clock lunge

The clock lunge is a variation to the normal lunge. Complete a forward lunge but instead of bring the leg into the starting position, take a step to the right and do another lunge. Place your feet behind you and perform a backward lunge. Return to the starting position and repeat the same moves on the other side.

Lunge jump

Lunge jump combines cardio and strength training. It can increase your heart rate while toning your legs. Bring your feet together and perform a lunge forward. Jump straight and drive your arms in front of you while keeping your elbows bent. Switch legs while in the air and land with the other leg forward. Continue to switch legs as you do several repetitions.

Side Kick

The side kick can target your leg and abdominal muscles. Start by placing your hands and knees on the floor. Keep your hands below your shoulders. Bend your knees in a 90-degree angle. Lift one leg until it is parallel to the floor. Kick the lifted leg to the side. Make sure not to lower your leg as you kick. Bend your knees and lower it to the starting position. Repeat on the other side.

Single leg balance touch

This exercise can challenge your balance. Stand on one leg and raise your arms over your head. Make sure that your spine is straight. Reach forward and bend you knee and you touch the ground. Squeeze your abs tight as you bend. Lower your other leg as you lift your arms overhead to finish the repetition. Don't forget to do the same exercise on the other leg.

Jump squat

This exercise is a plyometric exercise that can burn a lot of calories per minute. Start by positioning your body in a regular squat. Swing your arms behind you. Jump off the floor and swing both your arms to the ceiling. Land in the squat position and repeat.

High knee skips

High knee skip is inspired by a kid's game. Skip using one leg and drive it towards your chest. Make sure that the other leg is straight. Skip on the other leg to complete one repetition.

Pistol squat

Pistol squat is one of the most challenging squat variations. Extend your arms in front of you. Raise your right leg and drop down in a squat. Hold the position for a few seconds then straighten your legs. Repeat the movement on the other leg.

Chapter 4 Cardio Exercises

Cardio exercise always comes up in fitness and weight loss topics. Cardio is essential in maintaining a healthy body. Cardio exercise offers many physical and mental benefits.

Helps control weight

Cardio exercise is necessary if you want to lose weight. The total amount of calories burned will depend on intensity and duration. You do not need to work out for several hours to reap the benefits. Living an active lifestyle can also help you burn calories without going to the gym.

Combats health conditions

Cardio exercise can help reduce the risk of heart disease. Cardio exercise works the heart and lungs which can improve cardiovascular function. It can also improve blood cholesterol and triglyceride levels.

Improves your mood

Moderate exercise can help you feel better. Exercise can stimulate the production of endorphins that can make you feel more relaxed and reduce stress. Studies also show that people who regularly engage in cardio exercise have more confidence in their appearance. So, cardio can dramatically improve self esteem.

Increase the energy

One of the excuses that people use in avoiding cardio exercise is that they do not have enough energy. However, regular exercise can boost your endurance and increase your energy. Cardio exercise helps the body deliver oxygen and nutrients to the organs and tissues. This strengthens the lungs and heart, enabling you to have more energy to complete your chores.

Exercise promotes better sleep

Regular cardio exercise can improve your sleep. However, make sure that you do not exercise too close to bedtime since this can make you too energized to sleep.

Improves sex life

Regular cardio exercise can give you the energy and self-confidence to enjoy physical intimacy. Cardio exercise can also have positive effect on your sex life. It enhances arousal for women and reduces the risk of erectile dysfunction for men.

It is fun

Cardio exercise should not be boring. There are a lot of cardio exercises that can cater to different fitness levels. You can also enjoy cardio exercises with your family and friends.

Choosing your cardio exercise

Consider what kind of activities you enjoy. You should find activities that can fit your personality and something that you feel comfortable in. You can exercise indoors or outdoors. You can make your workout challenging by increasing its speed and intensity. Aim to perform cardio exercises three times in a week.

Duration

Beginners should start with 10-20 minutes of cardio exercise each day. You can gradually increase the time as you become more comfortable with the exercise. Most guidelines recommend at least 60 minutes of cardiovascular workout most days of the week.

If you feel that you cannot complete one hour workout straight, you can divide it into smaller workouts and spread it throughout the day. Also, it is important to make time for cardio exercises. People who exercise do not have more time than people that don't. They just learned how to make their health a priority. Schedule your workout and treat it just like any other appointment.

Frequency

The frequency of your workouts will depend on your lifestyle and fitness level. Most beginners find it comfortable to exercise for 3 non-consecutive days. If you want to lose weight, aim to work out 4 days in a week for at least 30 minutes each session. Athletes and people who are training for events, like triathlons, should work out most days of a week.

Remember that it will take some time for your body to build strength and endurance. Do not be disappointed if you cannot complete a rigorous workout the first time and keep trying.

Intensity

Once you are used to working out most days of the week, you can start adjusting your intensity. How hard you exercise is one of the most important factors in your work out since it is directly related to the amount of calories burned.

High intensity workout burns more calories per minute so it is great for people who don't have enough time to exercise. You can monitor your intensity with a heart rate monitor or by using a personal perceived exertion scale. A heart rate monitor is a device that gives you a continuous heart reading. Most heart rate monitors also measure calories burned and workout comparison. A perceived exertion scale is a measurement of intensity depending on a person's fitness level. Level 1 is a relaxed state, while level 10 is where you are exhausted and unable to continue the exercise anymore.

There are different levels of intensity and you can incorporate it in a single workout.

High intensity cardio can be described as 75-85% maximum heart rate. This could also be a level 7 or 8 in a perceived exertion scale. It is where you are sweating so much and find it difficult to talk. High intensity exercises can burn a lot of calories in just a short amount of time.

Moderate intensity cardio falls in 60-70% heart rate scale. It is where you can still talk but find it difficult to sing. Moderate intensity is often recommended in most exercise guides. This should be your target for most of your workouts.

Low intensity cardio can only increase your heart rate by 50-55%. It should be at level 3 or 4 in the perceived exertion scale. It is where you are still comfortable but may be breathing a little harder. Low intensity is a great level to work out at when you are warming up or cooling down.

Cardio Bodyweight Exercises

Bodyweight exercise can be a great way to increase heart rate without any special equipment.

Warm-up

Power skip

Skipping is not just a game for children. Start by standing with both of your feet apart. Raise your knee to your hips and skip. Land on your feet and repeat the same movement on the opposite leg. Aim to complete 10 skips on each leg.

High knees

High knee is a great way to warm up your muscles and strengthen your legs at the same time. Stand with your feet apart and lift your knees as high as you can go. Bring your leg down and alternate legs. Make sure that you do this exercise quickly. Aim to do this for 30 seconds at minimum.

Butt kick

Butt kick is a staple in many exercise circuits. Start gaining your momentum by jogging in place. Drive your heels towards your butt. The movement should be powered by the hamstring. Do not aimlessly kick your feet backwards. You can pick up the pace as you become comfortable.

Boxer's shuffle and switch

The boxer's shuffle can improve your speed and agility. Lift your hands in guard. Place your right foot in front of the left. Slightly bend your knees then switch to the other side by jumping. You should land with your left foot forward. Perform the exercise as quickly as you can.

Stair climb

The stair climb is great outdoor workout. You can even do it wherever there are stairs. Briskly walk up and down the stairs until your feel your body warming up. Travel the whole staircase and limit the amount of turns.

Inchworm

Start by standing tall. Lower your torso until your fingers touch the floor. Walk your hands forward. Make sure that you keep your feet straight. Keep walking your hands until you reach a push-up position. Walk your hands backward and straighten your body.

Jumping jacks

Jumping jacks is one of the classic exercise moves that can increase your heart rate dramatically. Make sure to keep your core engaged. Start with your feet wide apart. Jump your legs outward while raising your arms overhead. Slightly bend your knees as you jump to bring your feet together again.

Full body cardio exercises

Basic burpee

Burpees elicit a mixed emotion for people. It can be challenging for beginners but it targets the major muscle groups in the body. The jumping motion also increases the heart rate. Start in a squat position then extend your feet back in a push-up position. Drive your feet towards your chest and return to a squat position. Jump as high as you can before you squat low again.

Push-up burpee

The push-up burpee adds challenge to the basic burpee. You will have to do an actual push-up once you are in the plank position.

Single leg burpee

Once you have mastered the basic burpee, you can try this fancy variation. Complete a burpee but only use one leg. Switch to the other leg and repeat.

Long jump

The long jump is not reserved for the track and field team alone. Start by standing with your feet hips width apart. Jump and land on both legs at the same time. Aim to perform 10 repetitions in a row.

Vertical jump

The goal for the exercise is to jump as high as you can. Stand with your feet apart. Bend your knees slightly then propel your body upwards. Extend your arms overhead. Aim to complete 10 repetitions.

Invisible jump rope

You do not need an actual jump rope to do this exercise. Keep your feet together as you make small quick jumps. You should land at the balls of your feet. Place your hands to your side and make small movements as if you are holding a rope.

Frog jump

The frog jump can engage your entire body. Start in a squat position. Lower your torso and touch the floor with both of your hands. Make sure to keep your arms straight. Quickly jump and raise your knees high before you land.

Chapter 5 The Bodyweight Training Program

Here are two bodyweight training programs (one for each difficulty level):

<u>8-week Beginner Program</u>

This beginner workout program should be performed 3 days in a week. You can choose your workout days depending on your schedule. Be sure to rest in-between sessions.

- Week 1

Warm-up: (2 rounds)

Jog in place- 1 minute

Jumping jacks- 1 minute

High knees- 1 minute

Butt kicks- 1 minute

Jog in place- 1 minute

Exercise: (2 rounds)

Basic burpees- 12 reps

Vertical jump- 12 reps

Frog jumps- 12 reps

Russian Twist- 12 reps

Bicycle crunch- 15 reps

Squat- 15 reps

Wall sit- 12 reps

Lunge- 8 reps each leg

Cool-down: (2 rounds)

Slow jog- 1 minute

Inchworm- 1 minute

Wrist extensions- 1 minute

- Week 2

Perform this workout 3 days in week 2.

Warm-up: (2 rounds)

Power skip- 1 minute

High knees- 1 minute

Boxer's shuffle and twist- 1 minute

Butt kicks- 1 minute

Jumping jacks- 1 minute

Exercise: (2 rounds)

Plank- 4 reps, 20 seconds each

Side plank- 10 reps each side

Push-ups- 12 reps

Judo pushups- 12 reps

Reverse fly- 15 reps

Back-extensions- 12 reps

Chair dips- 12 reps

Decline push-ups- 12 reps

Lunge jumps- 8 reps per side

High knee skips- 12 reps

Cool down:

Jog in place- 2 minutes

Stretching

- Week 3

Warm-up (2 rounds)

Jog in place- 1 minute

Power skip- 1 minute

Jumping jacks- 1 minute

Stair climb- 1 minute

Inchworm- 1 minute

Exercise: (2 rounds)

Push-ups- 16 reps

Donkey kick- 16 reps

Side Plank- 10 reps each side

Skip twist- 16 reps

Knuckle push-up-16 reps

Power punch- 10 reps each side

Uppercut- 10 reps each side

Squat- 16 reps

Single balance touch- 10 reps each leg

Side kick- 10 reps each side

Cool down: (2 rounds)

Inchworm- 15 reps

The hip bridge- 1 minute

Stretching

- Week 4

Warm-up (2 rounds)

Jog in place- 2 minutes

Jumping jacks- 1 minute

Butt kicks- 1 minute

Exercise: (3 rounds)

Judo push-up- 8 reps

Dolphin push-ups- 8 reps

Bird dog exercise- 8 reps

Muscle-ups- 8 reps

Reverse push-ups

Burpees- 10 reps

Frog jump 10 reps

Jump squat- 10 reps

Cool down:

Invisible jump rope- 1 minute

Inchworms- 15 reps

Stretching

- Week 5

Warm-up: (3 rounds)

Power skip- 1 minute

Stair climb- 1 minute

Jumping jacks- 1 minute

Exercises: (3 rounds)

Push-up burpee-12 reps

Single leg burpee- 8 reps each leg

Frog jump- 12 reps

Reverse fly- 12 reps

Bird dog exercise- 12 reps

Bicycle crunch- 15 reps

Flutter kicks- 15 reps

Plank- 6 reps for 15 seconds each

Cool down:

Slow high knees- 1 minute

Slow butt kicks- 1 minute

Walk in place- 2 minutes

- Week 6

Warm-up: (3 rounds)

Jog in place- 1 minute

Jumping jacks- 1 minute

Butt kicks- 1 minute

Exercise: (3 rounds)

Frog jumps- 16 reps

Vertical jumps- 16 reps

Wrist curls- 16 reps

Power push-up- 16 reps

Wall-sit- 16 reps

Clock lunge- 16 reps

High knee skips- 16 reps

Towel wring-out- 1 minute

Cool down: (2 rounds)

Slow jumping jack- 1 minute

Jog in place- 1 minute

- Week 7

Warm-up: (3 rounds)

Jog in place- 1 minute

Quick high knees- 1 minute

Quick jumping jacks- 1 minute

Exercise: (3 rounds)

Burpees- 15 reps

Long jump- 15 reps

V- sit- 15 reps

Bicycle crunch- 15 reps

Skip twist- 15 reps

Single leg balance touch- 10 reps each leg

Side kick- 10 reps each leg

Wall sit- 16 reps

Wrist curls- 12 reps each arm

Hammer curl- 12 reps each arm

Cool down

Crab walk- 1 minute

Jumping jack- 1 minute

Inchworm- 1 minute

- Week 8

Warm- up: (3 rounds)

Jog in place- 1 minute

Jumping jacks- 1 minute

Butt kicks- 1 minute

Boxer's shuffle and switch- 1 minute

Exercise: (3 rounds)

Invisible jump rope- 1 minute

Donkey kicks- 16 reps

Reverse fly- 16 reps

Bird dog exercise- 16 reps

Sprinter sit-ups- 16 reps

Knuckle push-ups-16 reps

Archer pull-ups- 16 reps

Power punch- 12 reps each arm

Uppercut- 12 reps each arm

Hammer curl- 12 reps each arm

Cool down:

Jog in place- 2 minutes

Inchworm- 2 minutes

Stretching

8-Week Intermediate/Advanced Program

This intermediate/advanced program has more variety but it still challenges your body.

- Weeks 1 and 2

Choose one of the two circuits as your main workout. Perform each circuit twice in a week for a total of four workouts. For week two, increase the repetitions by 5.

Warm-up: (2 rounds)

Jog in place- 1 minute

Jumping jacks- 1 minute

Power skips- 1 minute

Circuit 1: Upper Body (3 rounds)

Burpees- 18- 23 reps

Push-ups- 18- 23 reps

Pike push-ups-18-23 reps

Judo push-ups-18-23 reps

Triceps extensions- 18-23 reps

Power punch- 15-20 reps each arm

Uppercut- 15-20 reps each arm

Circuit 2: Lower Body (3 rounds)

Long jump-18-23 reps

Russian twist- 18-23 reps

Sprinter sit-ups- 18-23 reps

Flutter kicks- 18-23 reps

Squat- 20-25 reps

Lunge- 20-25 reps

High knee skips- 18-23 reps

Cool down:

Jumping jacks- 1 minute

Inchworm- 1 minute

Stretching

- Weeks 3 and 4

Choose one circuit per day of workout. Aim to do each circuit twice in a week. Make sure that you alternate each circuit. Increase the repetitions by 5 for the fourth week.

Warm-up (3 rounds)

Jog in place- 1 minute

Butt kicks- 1 minute

Stair climb- 1 minute

Circuit 1: Upper body (3 rounds)

Frog jumps- 15-20 reps

Knuckle push-ups- 20-25 reps

Decline push-ups- 20-25 reps

Reverse fly- 20-25 reps

Crab walk- 15-20 reps

Hindu push-ups 20 -25 reps

Mountain climbers- 1 minute

Shoulder rotation- 15-20 reps per side

Wrist curls- 15-20 reps per arm

Towel wring out- 1 minute

Cool down:

Invisible jump rope- 1 minute

Inchworm- 1 minute

Hammer curl- 15-10 reps

- Weeks 5 and 6

Weeks 5 to 6 are challenging since you will be working out for 6 days in a week. Perform each circuit 3 times in a week. Increase the reps by 5 counts for week 6. These workouts can be completed in less than an hour.

Warm-up: (3 rounds)

Jog in place- 1 minute

Stair climb- 1 minute

High knees- 1 minute

Circuit 1: Upper Body (3 rounds)

Invisible jump rope- 1.5 minutes

Vertical jumps- 18-23 reps

Reverse push-ups- 18-23 reps

One arm push-ups- 18-23 reps

Donkey kick- 18-23 reps

Archer pull-ups- 18-23 reps

Skip twist- 20-25 reps

Alternating superman- 12-17 reps per side

Circuit 2: Lower body (3 rounds)

Single leg burpee- 18-23 reps

Frog jumps- 18-23 reps

Pistol squats- 12-17 reps each side

Jump squat- 18-23 reps

Side kick- 12-17 reps each side

Clock lunge- 18-23 reps

Flutter kicks- 18-23 reps

Bicycle crunch- 18-23 reps

Cool down:

Plank- 6 reps, 15 seconds each

Stretching

- Weeks 7 and 8

Perform each circuit thrice a week. Alternate the circuits to allow your muscles to rest.

Warm-up: (3 rounds)

Power skips- 1 minute

Butt kicks- 1 minute

Jumping jack- 1 minute

High knees- 1 minute

Circuit 1: Upper body (3 rounds)

Knuckle push-ups- 18-23 reps

Decline push-ups- 18-23 reps

Triceps extensions- 12-17 reps each arm

Handstand push-ups- 10-15 reps

Pike push-ups- 18-23 reps

Human flag- 45 seconds

Crab walk- 18-23 reps

Mountain climbers- 18-23 reps

Hip bridge- 18-23 reps

Side plank- 12-17 reps each side

Circuit 2: Lower body (3 rounds)

Long jump- 18-23 reps

Single leg burpee- 12-17 reps per side

Wall sits- 20-25 reps

Squats- 20-25 reps

Lunge jump- 18-23 reps

Pistol squats- 18-23 reps

Single leg balance touch- 12-17 reps per side

Lunge- 18-23 reps

Clock lunge- 18-23 reps

High knee skips- 18-23 reps

Cool down: (2 rounds)

Shoulder rotation- 15 reps

Wrist curls- 10 reps each arm

Hammer curl- 10 reps each arm

Conclusion

Thank you again for reading this book!   I hope this book was able to help you to do bodyweight exercises.

The next step is to try the 8-week program.

Finally, if you enjoyed this book, would you be kind enough to leave a review?

Thank you and good luck!

Mike

Additional Resources

Turbulence Training
http://www.deepthoughtpress.com/cardio-is-bad

Learn why the Wall Street Journal claims cardio is as bad as cheeseburgers and 3 other shocking facts about fat loss.

The Truth About Abs
http://www.deepthoughtpress.com/abs-truth

Uncover the truth about shrinking your stomach, melting away your stubborn stomach fat, and the 16 unusual, yet super –simple tips and tricks to keeping it off for good.

Take Control of Your Fitness with 101 Bodyweight Exercises
http://www.deepthoughtpress.com/101-exercises

This video course teach you 101 bodyweight exercises, 51 workout routines and 7 training protocols to create your own customized workouts.

Close Combat Fitness: Ultimate 15 Minute Bodyweight Workout
http://www.deepthoughtpress.com/combat-fitness

This video training course reveals the astonishing "accidental" workout discovery to getting strong, lean, and mean as fast as humanly possible.

Lose 53 Pounds in 6 weeks
http://www.deepthoughtpress.com/53-in-6

Learn the exact fat destroying method to melt off every last bit of fat of your body.   This method has been used by over 7,000 people. See the results for yourself.